THE OZEMPIC
Diet

Unveiling the Ozempic Diet's Blueprint for Lasting Weight Transformation

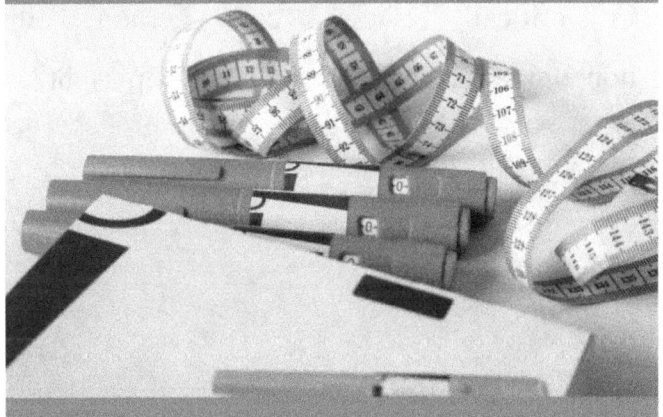

Dr. Irene M. Miller

Table of Contents

Chapter 1: Introduction to the Ozempic Diet ... 5

Chapter 2: Embarking on the Ozempic Diet Journey.............. 11

Chapter 3: Navigating the Nutritional Landscape 19

Chapter 4: Harnessing the Power of Exercise 25

Chapter 5: Leveraging Behavioral and Lifestyle Modifications.................. 33

Chapter 6: Optimizing Sleep and Overall Well-being 39

Chapter 7: Monitoring Progress and Adjusting Strategies 45

Chapter 8: Sustaining Results and Embracing a Healthy Lifestyle 51

Conclusion.................... 57

Chapter 1: Introduction to the Ozempic Diet

The Ozempic Diet is a weight control technique that combines the medicine Ozempic (semaglutide), a glucagon-like peptide-1 (GLP-1) receptor agonist, in conjunction with lifestyle adjustments such as diet and exercise. Ozempic is generally used to treat type 2 diabetes, but it has also shown potential in aiding weight loss.

How Ozempic Works

Ozempic works by imitating the actions of GLP-1, a hormone that helps manage blood sugar levels and hunger. When GLP-1 is released, it communicates to the brain to suppress hunger and increase fullness, resulting in reduced calorie intake. Ozempic also slows down gastric emptying, the rate at which food leaves the stomach, which further contributes to feelings of fullness.

Potential Benefits of the Ozempic Diet

Studies have shown that the Ozempic Diet can lead to significant weight loss, with individuals typically losing roughly 10-15% of their body weight over a year. Additionally, the Ozempic Diet has been connected with numerous health advantages, including:

• Improved blood sugar regulation

• Reduced blood pressure

• Lower cholesterol levels

• Enhanced insulin sensitivity

Science behind Ozempic and its impact on weight loss

The Ozempic Diet is founded on good scientific grounds. GLP-1, the hormone that Ozempic mimics, plays a critical function in controlling hunger and energy balance. Studies have demonstrated that GLP-1 receptor agonists, like Ozempic, can effectively suppress hunger and reduce food intake.

Clinical Studies on Ozempic and Weight Loss

Several clinical trials have tested the effectiveness of Ozempic in facilitating weight loss. A 2021 study published in the New England Journal of Medicine indicated that patients who got Ozempic lost much more weight than those who received a placebo.

Common misconceptions and concerns about the Ozempic Diet

Despite the positive studies, various myths and concerns surround the Ozempic Diet. Here are some popular questions and answers:

Is the Ozempic Diet safe?

Ozempic is generally safe and well-tolerated. However, some potential side effects include nausea, vomiting, diarrhea, and stomach pain. These side effects are often moderate and transient.

Is the Ozempic Diet a wonder pill?

No, the Ozempic Diet is not a miraculous medication. It is a weight management technique that requires lifestyle alterations such as food and exercise. Ozempic can be a helpful tool, but it is not a substitute for healthy practices.

Is the Ozempic Diet expensive?

Ozempic is a prescription drug, and its cost might vary based on insurance coverage. However, there are copay assistance programs available to help lower the expense.

Who is a good candidate for the Ozempic Diet?

The Ozempic Diet is suited for adults who are overweight or obese and have a body mass index (BMI) of 30 or higher. It may also be appropriate for persons with type 2 diabetes.

Important Considerations

Before starting the Ozempic Diet, it is vital to check with a healthcare practitioner to decide if it is right for you. They can help you assess your specific needs and build a personalized plan to attain your weight loss objectives.

Chapter 2: Embarking on the Ozempic Diet Journey

The Ozempic Diet, a weight management plan that combines the medicine Ozempic with lifestyle adjustments, offers a potential method to attaining sustainable weight loss. However, going on this journey involves considerable decision and preparation to ensure a successful and satisfying experience.

Assessing Suitability for the Ozempic Diet

Before considering the Ozempic Diet, it is vital to analyze whether it matches your individual demands and health situation.

Consulting with a healthcare professional is crucial to establish your suitability for this strategy. Your healthcare practitioner will assess your medical history, current medications, and overall health to determine if the Ozempic Diet is right for you.

Factors to Consider

During the assessment, your healthcare professional will evaluate numerous criteria, including:

• **Body mass index (BMI):** The Ozempic Diet is often suggested for persons with a BMI of 30 or higher, indicating obesity.

• **Underlying medical issues:** The presence of certain health disorders, such as type 2 diabetes, may make the Ozempic Diet a more viable alternative.

• **Current drugs:** Your healthcare professional will check your current medications to verify there are no potential interactions with Ozempic.

• **Individual tastes and lifestyle:** Your healthcare professional will examine your lifestyle patterns and preferences to adapt the Ozempic Diet plan accordingly.

Establishing Realistic Weight Loss Goals and Expectations

Setting realistic weight reduction goals is vital for keeping motivation and preventing discouragement during the Ozempic Diet journey. Healthcare practitioners propose setting modest and manageable objectives, aiming for a weight loss of 1-2 pounds per week.

Understanding Your Weight Loss Potential

The Ozempic Diet can effectively stimulate weight loss, often leading to a loss of roughly 10-15% of body weight over a year. However, individual results may vary depending on factors such as beginning weight, adherence to the diet plan, and overall lifestyle adjustments.

Managing Expectations

Remember that the Ozempic Diet is a journey, not a fast fix. Expecting rapid or substantial weight loss might lead to disappointment and anger. Instead, focus on incremental growth and enjoy your victories along the way.

Creating a Personalized Ozempic Diet Plan

A bespoke Ozempic Diet plan should be adapted to your unique needs, interests, and lifestyle. This strategy should contain a combination of food adjustments, activity advice, and Ozempic drug supervision.

Dietary Modifications

The Ozempic Diet primarily stresses a balanced and healthful eating pattern, emphasizing whole foods, fruits, vegetables, and lean protein sources. Limiting processed foods, sugary drinks, and extra harmful fats is vital for attaining weight loss goals.

Exercise Recommendations

Regular physical activity plays a key role in weight management and general health. Aim for at least 150 minutes of moderate-intensity aerobic exercise or 75 minutes of vigorous-intensity aerobic exercise every week. Incorporate strength training workouts at least twice a week to build muscle mass, which boosts metabolism and encourages fat burning.

Ozempic Medication Guidance

Your healthcare practitioner will establish the optimum amount and frequency of Ozempic administration depending on your unique needs. It is vital to follow the specified drug regimen and attend regular follow-up consultations to monitor your progress and make adjustments as needed.

Embark on Your Ozempic Diet Journey with Confidence

With careful preparation, individualized planning, and continued assistance from your healthcare professional, you can confidently embark on the Ozempic Diet journey.

Remember, persistence and perseverance are crucial to attaining sustained weight loss and increasing your entire health and well-being.

Chapter 3: Navigating the Nutritional Landscape

The core of the Ozempic Diet rests in adopting a balanced and nutritious eating pattern. This strategy stresses ingesting complete, unprocessed meals that supply key nutrients for good health and help sustainable weight loss.

Key Principles of Balanced Nutrition

• **Variety:** Consume a varied range of foods from all food groups, including fruits, vegetables, whole grains, lean protein sources, and healthy fats.

- **Moderation:** Practice mindful eating and portion control to avoid overconsumption.

- **Balance:** Aim to attain a balance of macronutrients - carbohydrates, proteins, and healthy fats – to meet your body's energy needs and support general health.

- **Nutrient Density:** Choose nutrient-rich foods that supply necessary vitamins, minerals, and phytonutrients for maximum health and well-being.

Implementing Ozempic Diet-Friendly Meal Plans and Recipes

Crafting Ozempic Diet-friendly meal planning and recipes is vital for success. Here are some recommendations for producing nutritious and pleasant meals that accord with the concepts of balanced nutrition:

• **Plan Ahead:** Plan your meals for the week to minimize last-minute bad choices.

• **Stock Your Pantry:** Keep your pantry stocked with nutritious essentials, such as whole grains, fresh fruits and vegetables, lean protein sources, and healthy fats.

• **Embrace Flavorful Cooking:** Explore new recipes and cooking techniques to make healthy meals more enticing.

• **Incorporate Ozempic Friendly Substitutions** : Replace high-calorie foods with healthy alternatives, such as using whole-wheat bread instead of white bread or using low-fat dairy products.

• **Seek Inspiration:** Utilize online resources, cookbooks, and meal-planning apps for inspiration and assistance.

Managing Cravings and Making Mindful Food Choices

Cravings can represent a big obstacle when trying to maintain a balanced diet. Here are some techniques to properly manage urges and make mindful meal choices:

• **Identify Craving Triggers:** Recognize the situations, emotions, or times of day that often cause cravings.

• **Distract Yourself:** Engage in activities that divert your focus from urges, such as going for a stroll, listening to music, or participating in a pastime.

- **Address Emotional Eating:** Seek healthy coping techniques for stress and emotional triggers, such as exercise, meditation, or journaling.

- **Practice Mindful Eating:** Pay attention to hunger cues, eat deliberately, and savor each meal to increase satisfaction and minimize overeating.

- **Plan for Cravings:** Keep healthy snacks available to fulfill cravings when they emerge, such as fruit, veggies, almonds, or yogurt.

Remember, the Ozempic Diet is not about deprivation but rather about choosing informed and mindful eating choices that support your weight reduction objectives and overall well-being.

Chapter 4: Harnessing the Power of Exercise

Regular physical exercise is a key component of the Ozempic Diet, combining synergistically with medicine and dietary adjustments to promote weight loss, boost general health, and improve well-being.

The Benefits of Exercise

Exercise plays a significant part in weight management:

• **Increasing calorie expenditure:** Physical activity burns calories, providing a calorie deficit that leads to weight loss.

- **Building and maintaining muscle mass:** Muscle mass enhances metabolism, helping the body burn more calories even at rest.

- **Enhancing insulin sensitivity:** Exercise enhances the body's capacity to use insulin, the hormone that regulates blood sugar levels.

- **Promoting general health:** Regular exercise reduces the risk of chronic diseases such as heart disease, stroke, type 2 diabetes, and some types of cancer.

Incorporating Exercise into Your Routine

Aim for at least 150 minutes of moderate-intensity aerobic exercise or 75 minutes of vigorous-intensity aerobic exercise every week. Spread your exercise throughout the week, aiming for at least 30 minutes of moderate-intensity activity most days.

Choosing Appropriate Exercise Types

Select activities that you enjoy and can sustain over time. Consider a range of workouts to target different muscle areas and keep your program entertaining. Here are several examples:

- **Aerobic exercise:** Brisk walking, jogging, swimming, cycling, dancing

- **Strength training:** Weightlifting, bodyweight exercises, resistance bands

- **Mind-body exercises:** Yoga, Pilates, tai chi

Intensity Levels

Moderate-intensity exercise should boost your heart rate and respiration, but you should still be able to carry on a conversation. Vigorous-intensity exercise makes it harder to maintain a conversation.

Overcoming Exercise Barriers

Starting and keeping a fitness routine can be tough. Here are some techniques to overcome typical barriers:

• **Set realistic goals:** Start with achievable goals and progressively raise the intensity and duration of your workouts.

• **Schedule workouts:** Treat exercise like an essential appointment and set out time in your schedule.

• **Find an exercise buddy**: Having a workout companion can bring inspiration and accountability.

• **Make it enjoyable:** Choose activities you find pleasant and intriguing.

• **Start slowly:** Begin with shorter, less difficult workouts and gradually increase as your fitness improves.

• **Track your success:** Keep a record of your workouts to monitor your progress and stay inspired.

Staying Motivated

Maintaining motivation can be challenging, especially in the long haul. Here are some methods to keep oneself motivated:

• **Focus on the benefits:** Remind yourself of the wonderful influence of exercise on your weight loss, health, and overall well-being.

• **Celebrate your achievements:** Acknowledge and praise yourself for reaching milestones and maintaining consistency.

• **Discover a supportive community:** Join a fitness class, or online forum, or discover people with similar aspirations.

• **Don't be scared to modify:** Adjust your training program as needed to avoid injury or boredom.

• **Seek inspiration:** Read success stories, watch motivational movies, or listen to motivating podcasts.

Remember, consistency is crucial to getting the benefits of exercise. Find strategies to make physical activity a joyful and sustainable part of your lifestyle.

Chapter 5: Leveraging Behavioral and Lifestyle Modifications

Achieving sustainable weight loss using the Ozempic Diet demands not only food and exercise improvements but also addressing underlying behavioral habits that may inhibit achievement. Identifying and comprehending these tendencies is vital for establishing successful tactics to overcome them.

Common Behavioral Patterns that Hinder Weight Loss

• **Emotional Eating:** Using food to cope with stress, worry, or boredom

- **Mindless Eating:** Eating without consciousness, frequently owing to distractions or emotional impulses

- **Rewarding Yourself with Food:** Associating food with rewards or celebrations

- **All-or-Nothing Thinking:** Labeling yourself as "good" or "bad" based on dietary choices

- **Lack of Self-Compassion:** Criticizing yourself severely for losses or perceived failures

Strategies for Addressing Behavioral Patterns

- **Identify Triggers:** Recognize situations, feelings, or times of day that frequently contribute to poor eating practices.

- **Develop Healthy Coping Mechanisms:** Find alternate ways to manage stress, worry, or boredom, such as exercise, meditation, or journaling.

- **Practice Mindful Eating:** Pay attention to hunger cues, eat deliberately, and savor each meal to increase satisfaction and minimize overeating.

• **Challenge All-or-Nothing Thinking:** Replace negative thinking with more balanced and realistic self-talk.

• **Embrace Self-Compassion:** Acknowledge setbacks as part of the learning process and practice self-kindness.

Developing Healthy Lifestyle Habits

Incorporating healthy lifestyle practices beyond diet and exercise is vital for long-term success with the Ozempic Diet and general well-being.

• **Prioritize Quality Sleep:** Aim for 7-8 hours of quality sleep each night to regulate hormones, enhance metabolism, and improve mood.

• **Manage Stress Effectively:** Practice stress-reduction strategies such as yoga, meditation, or deep breathing to maintain emotional balance and minimize stress-related eating.

• **Maintain a Regular pattern:** Establish a constant daily pattern that includes regular meals, exercise, and sleep to enhance stability and prevent impulsive decisions.

• **Surround Yourself with Support:** Build a supportive network of family, friends, or a healthcare professional to provide encouragement and accountability.

• **Maintain a Positive Mindset:** Cultivate a positive mindset and focus on progress rather than perfection.

Remember, behavioral and lifestyle adjustments are not only about changing habits; they are about creating a healthier and more rewarding connection with food and your entire well-being.

Chapter 6: Optimizing Sleep and Overall Well-being

Sleep has a critical role in weight management, overall health, and well-being. When sleep is disrupted, hormones that govern appetite and metabolism become imbalanced, leading to increased hunger and cravings and decreased energy expenditure. Aim for 7-8 hours of excellent sleep each night to gain the benefits of adequate sleep for weight loss and overall health.

Establish a Consistent Sleep Schedule

• **Set Regular Sleep Times:** Go to bed and wake up at consistent times each day, especially on weekends, to control your body's natural sleep-wake cycle.

• **Create a Relaxing Bedtime Routine:** Wind down in the hour before bed by engaging in peaceful activities such as reading, having a warm bath, or listening to soothing music.

• **Avoid Stimulants Before Bed:** Avoid caffeine, alcohol, and electronic gadgets in the hours preceding up to sleep, as these might interfere with sleep quality.

• **Optimize Your Sleep Environment:** Create a dark, calm, and cool sleep environment to encourage healthy sleep.

Prioritize Quality Rest

• **Practice Sleep Hygiene:** Maintain correct sleep hygiene practices, such as avoiding daytime naps and resting for extended periods, to maximize nighttime sleep.

• **Address Sleep Issues:** If you experience sleep disruptions such as insomnia or sleep apnea, speak with a healthcare expert for diagnosis and treatment.

Practicing Stress-Reduction Techniques and Promoting Relaxation

Chronic stress can greatly hamper weight loss efforts by raising stress hormones that increase fat storage and reduce insulin sensitivity. Incorporating stress-reduction practices into your daily routine can help manage stress, enhance sleep quality, and boost general well-being.

• **Mindfulness and Meditation:** Practice mindfulness techniques such as meditation or deep breathing exercises to calm the mind, reduce stress, and promote relaxation.

• **Yoga and Tai Chi:** Engage in mind-body practices like yoga or tai chi to integrate physical activity with stress reduction, enhancing flexibility, balance, and overall well-being.

• **Indulging hobbies and things:** Pursue things that bring you joy and relaxation, whether it's reading, listening to music, spending time in nature, or indulging in creative hobbies.

• **Seek Social Connection:** Nurture strong social relationships and spend quality time with loved ones to reduce stress and boost emotional well-being.

Nurturing Overall Well-being for Sustainable Weight Management

Sustainable weight control extends beyond diet, exercise, and sleep; it entails establishing a holistic approach to total well-being.

• **Prioritize Physical Health:** Engage in regular physical activity, keep a balanced diet, and attend frequent check-ups with your healthcare practitioner.

• **Nurture Mental Health:** Practice mindfulness techniques, seek professional help when needed, and engage in activities that enhance emotional well-being.

• **Cultivate Self-Compassion:** Practice self-acceptance, avoid harsh self-criticism, and applaud your progress, no matter how tiny.

• **Seek Support:** Build a solid support system of family, friends, or a healthcare professional to provide encouragement and accountability.

Remember, sustainable weight management is a journey, not a destination. Prioritizing overall well-being, including proper sleep, stress management, and holistic self-care, is vital for long-term success in achieving your weight reduction objectives.

Chapter 7: Monitoring Progress and Adjusting Strategies

Regularly monitoring your weight loss journey

and reviewing your success is vital for keeping motivated, recognizing areas for growth, and making any adjustments to your Ozempic Diet plan.

Establish a Monitoring System

• **Choose a Tracking Method:** Select a method that meets your preferences, such as using a scale, measuring tape, or body composition monitor.

• **Set a Regular Schedule:** Weigh oneself at consistent times, for as once a week in the morning after using the restroom and before eating.

• **Track Additional Metrics:** Monitor other health indicators besides weight, such as body measurements, blood pressure, blood sugar levels (if appropriate), and overall energy levels.

• **Maintain a Progress notebook:** Keep a notebook to record your weight, measurements, observations, and any adjustments you make to your food or exercise program.

Evaluating Progress

• **Focus on Long-term Trends:** Avoid getting disheartened by short-term swings in weight. Instead, focus on broad trends over time.

• **Celebrate Milestones:** Acknowledge and celebrate your victories, no matter how minor, to retain motivation and reinforce positive behavior changes.

• **Find Areas for Improvement:** Analyze your progress journal and find areas where you may need to make adjustments, such as increasing exercise intensity or making nutritional modifications.

Identifying Areas for Improvement and Making Adjustments to Your Ozempic Diet Plan

As you evaluate your progress, you may need to make adjustments to your Ozempic Diet plan to optimize outcomes and handle any obstacles.

• **Assess Dietary Habits:** Evaluate your food choices, portion sizes, and adherence to the Ozempic Diet guidelines.

• **Analyze Exercise Routine:** Review your exercise frequency, intensity, and kind to verify it corresponds with your goals and development.

• **Consider Underlying Variables:** Identify any underlying variables that may be influencing your success, such as stress, sleep quality, or prescription interactions.

• **Consult with Your Healthcare Provider:** Seek help from your healthcare provider to make educated adjustments to your Ozempic Diet plan, medication dosage, or overall approach.

Seeking Support from a Healthcare Professional When Needed

Throughout your Ozempic Diet journey, don't hesitate to get support from your healthcare provider when needed.

- **Regular Check-ups:** Attend regular follow-up appointments with your healthcare practitioner to monitor your progress, discuss any issues, and make appropriate modifications.

- **Addressing obstacles:** Seek advice if you find obstacles, such as plateaus, cravings, or difficulty adhering to the diet plan.

- **Managing Side Effects:** Discuss any side effects connected with Ozempic medicine and seek alternate treatment alternatives if necessary.

- **Tailored Advice:** Receive individualized advice and support tailored to your unique requirements, preferences, and health status.

Chapter 8: Sustaining Results and Embracing a Healthy Lifestyle

As you achieve your weight loss objectives with the Ozempic Diet, the question arises of moving off Ozempic and sustaining long-term success. This shift needs careful planning, sustained devotion to healthy behaviors, and a lifelong dedication to well-being.

Gradual Tapering Off Ozempic

Under the advice of your healthcare practitioner, you will gradually taper off Ozempic to prevent rebound weight gain. This approach entails gently lowering the medicine dosage over some time.

Maintaining Healthy Habits

The key to lasting weight loss rests in incorporating the good behaviors you've adopted during the Ozempic Diet into your daily routine. This includes:

• **Balanced and Nutritious Eating**: Continue making healthy food choices and keeping a balanced diet that delivers necessary nutrients for maximum health.

• **Regular Exercise:** Maintain a regular exercise plan that matches your tastes and fitness level. Aim for at least 150 minutes of moderate-intensity aerobic exercise or 75 minutes of vigorous-intensity aerobic exercise every week.

• **Mindful Eating:** Practice mindful eating to increase satiety, prevent overeating, and make thoughtful food choices.

• **Stress Management:** Continue using stress-reduction tactics to reduce stress levels and prevent stress-related eating.

• **Adequate Sleep:** Prioritize quality sleep by establishing a consistent sleep schedule and adopting a pleasant nighttime ritual.

• **Self-Compassion:** Cultivate self-compassion and avoid harsh self-criticism. Recognize that setbacks are part of the process and learn from them.

Cultivating a Lifelong Commitment to Health and Well-being

Sustainable weight control and overall well-being are not destinations but rather lifetime journeys. Here are some tips to keep a healthy lifestyle:

• **Continuous Learning:** Stay knowledgeable on nutrition, exercise, and overall well-being. Attend workshops, study books, or follow trustworthy internet resources.

• **Find Joy in Movement:** Discover physical activities that you enjoy and incorporate them into your routine.

• **Make Healthy Choices Convenient:** Stock your pantry with healthy snacks and prepare nutritious meals in advance to make healthy choices convenient.

• **Build a Support Network:** Surround yourself with supportive friends, family members, or a healthcare professional who can encourage and motivate you.

• **Seek Professional Help When Needed:** Don't hesitate to seek professional guidance from a registered nutritionist, a certified personal trainer, or a mental health expert when needed.

Remember, successful weight management is not about perfection but about making regular and conscious decisions that promote your overall health and well-being.

Conclusion

As you end your Ozempic Diet journey, take a minute to reflect on the wonderful transformation you have undergone. Acknowledge the hurdles you have overcome, the good habits you have formed, and the substantial progress you have made toward your weight reduction and well-being goals.

Celebrate Your Milestones

Take delight in every milestone you have attained along the way. Whether it's meeting a weight target, boosting your fitness level, or having a healthy relationship with food, each accomplishment deserves recognition and celebration.

Embrace a Renewed Sense of Self-Confidence and Improved Health

The Ozempic Diet has not only altered your physical look but has also created in you a renewed feeling of self-confidence and an appreciation for your general health. Embrace this increased vitality and take it forward into every facet of your life.

Sharing Your Experiences and Inspiring Others to Achieve Their Wellness Goals

Your Ozempic Diet experience has surely been a source of personal growth and inspiration. Share your experiences, ideas, and newfound knowledge with others to empower them to embark on their wellness journeys.

Become a Beacon of Hope and Encouragement

Your achievement can act as a light of hope and inspiration for others wanting to better their health and well-being. Share your story openly and honestly, offering encouragement and assistance to people who may be battling with their weight reduction objectives.

Inspire Positive Change

Your journey can inspire good change in the lives of others, inspiring them to adopt healthier lifestyles and embrace a holistic approach to well-being.

Remember, the Ozempic Diet is not only about reducing weight; it's about obtaining a healthier, happier, and more confident version of yourself. As you move forward, continue to cultivate the healthy habits you've acquired and embrace the transformational potential of a healthy lifestyle.